Random Acts to

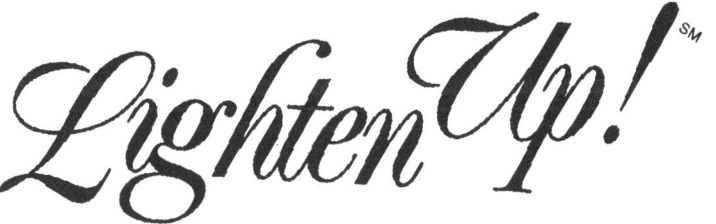

by Katie Evans

KENDALL/HUNT PUBLISHING COMPANY
4050 Westmark Drive   Dubuque, Iowa 52002

Cover design by Maestri, Seattle, WA

Back cover photograph by Julie Hanich, Seattle, WA

Copyright © 1997 by Katie Evans

ISBN 0-7872-4381-7

All rights reserved. No part of this publication may be reproduced, stored in a retrieval system, or transmitted, in any form or by any means, electronic, mechanical, photocopying, recording, or otherwise, without the prior written permission of the copyright owner.

Printed in the United States of America
10   9   8   7   6   5   4   3   2   1

This book is lovingly dedicated to

Cassandra, Stephany, and Rob.

"You are the light of the world. A city built on a hilltop cannot be hidden. No one lights a lamp to put it under a tub; they put it on the lampstand where it shines for everyone in the house. In the same way your light must shine in the sight of men, so that, seeing your good works, they may give the praise to your Father in heaven."
— Matthew 5:14-16

ACKNOWLEDGMENTS

I am a compilation of the people who love me. God has blessed me with you. You have contributed to the Lighten Up! vision in your own unique and indispensable ways and I love you.

Nan Bolomey, whose love and good sense and patience repeatedly keep me from tipping over.

Kathleen Campbell, always here to keep me in touch with my Source.

Rejeana Hartzell, who just *does it* every day.

Niki Young, who took Lighten Up! to a bigger playing field.

Lisa Crunick, whose dependability allows me the freedom to fly.

Joel Junker, my friend, my mentor, my brother, and the left side of my brain.

I would especially like to thank the thousands of Lighten Up! students who inspire me every day with your courage, willingness, and success. God Bless You!

PREFACE

Random Acts to Lighten Up! is the culmination of over 10 years of helping people successfully lose weight. I've discovered that there are no hard and fast rules to weight loss. "Rules" often create resistance and rebellion which can result in overeating. Different methods work for different people. I've included many suggestions in this book for you to *try*. It is not my intention to overload your already full life with more concepts to remember or things to do. Just play with some of the ideas presented here. You may enjoy the experiences and be pleased with the results.

This book is meant to be read differently than you may be used to reading. It's not to be read cover-to-cover. Instead, keep it with you and refer to it frequently. I recommend picking it up periodically, opening it to any page and begin reading. Almost invariably, you will read exactly what will help you most at that moment.

Lighten Up! has very little to do with your weight. It's more about your attitude. Weight has been far too "heavy" a subject for too long. When you begin to *Lighten Up!* your life, your body will follow.

This is a book about "baby steps." I believe that many small behaviors are easy to change and that they can lead to larger behavior changes. Remember to give yourself many pats on your own back for each small success. Whenever you move, however slightly, in the direction of your goals, it's good enough for now.

One of the most difficult activities for human beings to do is **think new thoughts**. Much of what you will read in this book will ask that you do just that: think about things in new and different ways. Aren't you getting bored thinking about the same old stuff in the same old ways? Let's have some fun with that gray matter!

Throughout this book you will see the symbol **Å** followed by a sentence. These sentences are affirmations. After you read one you may want to close your eyes for a moment and repeat it to yourself a few times. This can begin to redirect your mind to a more positive outlook.

There are several spaces throughout this book for you to write your thoughts or answer questions. Please take the time to do these exercises. Writing helps convert thoughts and ideas into behaviors.

I have very good news for you. Everything you do, you *learned* how to do. All behavior begins as *functional* behavior. That is, it worked for you at the time you learned it. What behaviors do you still have that aren't working for you any longer? Since all behavior is learned behavior, maybe it's just time to learn some new and more adaptive behaviors and skills.

I have many goals for you as you read this book: to inspire you to laugh, to feel, to cogitate, to learn new, healthier behaviors, and to experience "Aha's." Watch for the "Aha's." They'll sneak up on you and they're great fun!

To find out where Lighten Up! is being taught in your area, please call me: 1-888-763-5444 or e-mail me: *103755.1330@compuserve.com*. Visit our home page at *http://www.accessone.com/health/*

I sincerely hope that you enjoy reading this book and that it takes you on a path of self-discovery that never ends.

Katie Evans

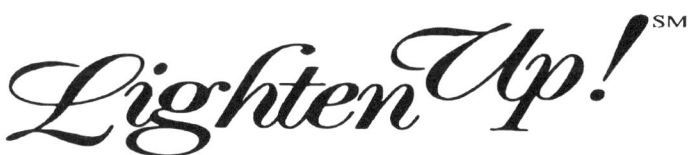
Lighten Up!^{SM}

Your stomach is the size of your fist—that's **pre-chewed food**! Today, look at your fist **before** eating anything. You'll be amazed how little food your body needs.

Whenever you have the urge to eat, stop just for a few seconds and ask yourself: "What am I really feeling?" If it's hunger, then eat. If the answer turns out to be "bored, angry, lonely," or any other feeling besides hunger, do whatever **really** makes you feel better.

If you really want conversation, for example, all the ice cream in the world is not going to satisfy you.

> *You can never get enough of what you really don't want.*
> — Dr. Wayne Dyer

Every second is the beginning of your life.

·· o ··

Å   *I trust the process of life.*

Don't worry about doing anything for the rest of your life. Just take care of today and tomorrow will take care of itself.

Stay present. Stay conscious.

To get in touch with your own inner power ***immediately***, ask yourself the following:

1. What is happening in my life that I don't want to happen?
2. What can I do about it?
3. Am I doing it?

> *No great thing is created suddenly,*
> *Any more than a bunch of grapes or a fig.*
> *If you tell me that you desire a fig.*
> *I answer you that there must be time.*
> *Let it first blossom, then bear fruit,*
> *Then ripen.*
> — Epicetetus

Breathe!

The three things necessary to burn fat are: heat, oxygen, and fat.

Nothing tastes as good as thin feels (and doesn't last nearly as long!).

Å *I take great pride in my appearance and I am always well-groomed.*

One of the primary functions of your brain is to maintain your sanity. How is being overweight and/or overeating keeping you sane?

Your subconscious mind will solve your problems for you the best way it can in the absence of instruction from you and it will almost always sacrifice your body to save your mind.

Your body will never lie to you, but your mind will lie all day long. It'll tell you things like, "There's just one piece of pie left in the kitchen. Let's eat it, then it will be gone, then we don't have to think about it anymore." So you do and about five minutes later, your mind yells, "What did you do that for?"

─────────── o ───────────

Everyone has their own version of the truth. If five people see a car accident, they'll give five different versions of what happened. If they all took a lie detector test, they'd all pass it! Knowledge of this simple fact will save you lots of time trying to convince others that they're wrong and you're right.

─────────── o ───────────

Not eating when you're hungry leads to overeating. It's as harmful as overeating. It doesn't take long for your body to go into deprivation.

Not eating when you're hungry leads to your body distrusting you. So when you finally do it, it's gonna "stock up" cause it's not sure when you're gonna feed it again!

> *If you think you can or you think you can't, you're right.*
>
> — Henry Ford

Replace the word "can't" in your conversation with "choose not to." Eliminate the word "try" all together.

> *There is no "try," there is only "do" or "don't do."*
> *— Master Yoda*

The whiter the bread, the quicker you're dead.

Å ***I enjoy spending quiet time with myself.
I find it fulfilling and relaxing.***

.... o ....

When someone gives you a compliment, say, "Thank you." Period. With no story—you know the things we say to invalidate the compliment—either to yourself or out loud.

Å ***I speak proper English at all times.***

Å ***I always remember names easily.***

.... o ....

Close your eyes, take a deep breath in, and imagine your metabolism. Some people imagine it as a car, train, horse, fireplace—anything that shows motion. Now speed it up. You may feel a warmth in your body. That's thermogenesis—creating heat (one of the things needed to burn fat!).

List 5 things in your life over which you have control:

1. _____

2. _____

3. _____

4. _____

5. _____

List 5 things in your life over which you have no control but think you do:

1. _____

2. _____

3. _____

4. _____

5. _____

MOVE YOUR BODY

Our bodies were built to move. If God hadn't meant for our bodies to move, they would look like big, heavy, steel boxes and they'd just sit there. Here are some easy ways to incorporate more movement into your life:

- Get rid of the remote controls in your life. (Okay, you're not going to do that. So just don't use them *all* the time!)
- Get together with others at work and walk before or after lunch.
- Don't *let* the dog out; *take* the dog out.
- One of my students lost 30 pounds in 4 months by changing just one behavior: he parked a mile away from work and walked the rest of the way.

Every movement you make has a cumulative effect on increasing your metabolism.

- If you ride the bus, get off two stops ahead of yours and walk the rest of the way.
- Speed up your pace when you walk. (Walk faster.)
- When you go to the mall, pick a place to park farthest from the entrance. Walk briskly to the door.
- Swing your arms when you walk.
- Take the stairs whenever possible. If you work on the 35th floor, take the elevator to the 30th floor and walk the rest of the way.

> *The way to develop self-confidence is to do the thing you fear and get a record of successful experiences behind you.*
> — William Jennings Bryan

You are emotionally attached to your body. So if you **hate** it, you're really stuck to it. Try respecting it (liking it may be too big a stretch right now). After all, for all the abuse you've heaped on it, it's still carrying you around!

Å ***I look so beautiful and sophisticated wearing all my new clothes. I am very sensual.***

○ ○ ○ ○ ○ ○ ○ ○

To relax quickly, make your belly soft and your jaw slack and drop your shoulders.

Breathe (breathing is our friend!)

―――――――――――――○―――――――――――――

Write one goal (affirmation) 15 times a day until you get it.

―――――――――――――○―――――――――――――

Å ***When I really trust that I'll take care of myself, I can let go enough to soar.***

If you have children, **take** them out to play instead of sending them out. Pretend it's recess for *you*.

Imagine yourself as a child when play (moving your body) was fun. Get in touch with the feelings of freedom and joy and motion.

Imagine what your life would be like with no limitations . . .

If you don't have children, borrow one for a day. Watch how they eat. They don't care what time it is or when dinner will be served. They're so in touch with their bodies, their hunger right now is all that matters. Learn from kids.

SAUTÉED SPINACH:

1 bunch fresh spinach
1 clove chopped garlic *or*
¼ tsp crushed garlic

Clean spinach thoroughly. Sauté (hot) in Pam™ with garlic. Stir rapidly for just a few minutes until spinach wilts and becomes hot. Serve immediately.

Ask your supermarket manager to stock any foods recommended here. That's how we get healthy food mainstreamed.

- For chocolate cravings, get Wax Orchards Fudge Sweet™. Zap a small amount in the microwave for 3 to 4 seconds. Dip banana, apple, pear. Decadent! And no refined sugar or fat!

- Take 200 mcg. chromium picolinate daily. It may cut your sugar cravings and help in the formation of lean muscle tissue when you exercise.

- Have one meatless day a week. It gives your body a rest and helps the planet.

- Eat a bite of protein with everything you eat. For some, it will cut your food cravings drastically.

- Shop on the outskirts of the supermarket. Most of the products located in the aisles are processed, sugar-laden and unnecessary (except toilet paper).

- Use Bragg's Liquid Aminos™ instead of soy sauce; it's better for you and contains less sodium.

Cravings for salty food (or salt-then-sugar cravings) usually means you're thirsty. Drink water.

- Get a water filter.

Mix herbal tea with juice. For example, cranberry tea and apple juice, orange spice tea with orange juice; mix 50-50.

··· o ···

Pay attention to the people in your life who try to "feed" you. Politely refrain.

Learn to say "no." It's the easiest and hardest word in the English language: Hard to learn and life gets *sssoooo* easy when you do!

··· o ···

Listen for when you say "I deserve." It usually means you're about to do something fattening, unhealthy, or too expensive!

Realize that you deserve love and food is not love, even though you don't have to shave your legs on a Saturday to have a "date" with a pizza!

Whatever it is, "Don't eat about it."

₀ ° ○ ○ ○ ○ ° ° °

You know you're eating enough fiber when your poop floats.

You know you're drinking enough water when your urine is clear, unless you're taking B and C vitamins—or eating asparagus!

Thorough preparation makes its own luck.
— Joe Poyer

Many overweight people are "rescuers," that is, they would rather help others than take care of themselves.

The nicest people—next to cancer patients—are overweight people. They deny their own needs and just eat instead.

There's a high positive correlation between cancer and unexpressed anger.

○

Make a conscious decision to abstain from one temptation for a day or an hour or whatever length of time you can manage. Do the best you can.

Know that you always do the best you can—if you **could** have done better, you **would** have done better.

> *Every man is free to rise*
> *as far as he's able or willing,*
> *but the degree to which he thinks*
> *determines the degree*
> *to which he'll rise*
>
> — Ayn Rand

Eliminate the "shouldas, wouldas, and couldas" from your vocabulary. They mainly serve to produce guilt.

Give yourself frequent pats on the back for making healthier choices.

GLORIOUS BATH SALTS:

1 box Epsom salts
3 drops of your favorite fragrance of essential oil
3 drops of your favorite food coloring

Put everything into a clear plastic bag and squish it all together until the color is even. Place into a lovely decanter in the bathroom. You can buy inexpensive decanters at a thrift store. Use as needed. These make great gifts, too!

Tell yourself the truth to the best of your ability.

Å *I am now willing to change and accept my personal growth. I leave the past behind me.*

- Wean yourself off caffeine gradually. Begin by drinking ¾ cup caf-¼ cup decaf. Gradually move to more decaf.

Nutrasweet® is 200 times sweeter than sugar.

- Take a workshop on building healthy boundaries. They are often offered through evening education programs at your local community colleges. It's also a great way to meet new people.

---o---

You can't attribute motivation to others. Your boss may yell at you not because you're a horrible person, but because her husband left her that morning.

---o---

Buy fresh flowers for yourself. Throw them away before they're all dead.

> **TERIYAKI POACHED SALMON**
>
> Place a salmon filet into a shallow pan of barely boiling water. Cook 4 to 6 minutes (until flaky). Remove from pan onto plate, cover with Bragg's Liquid Aminos.™ Fabulous!

Become a love finder rather than a fault finder.

Å   *I love to listen to my affirmations and do so every day.*

Watch how much you judge yourself and others. Don't judge your observations. Develop an "attitude of gratitude." Say "thank you" often.

Do what you love and love what you do. If you don't, either change your life or change your mind.

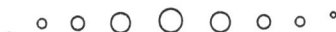

Pray with your feet moving.

Apply this to your life:

> *God grant me the serenity to accept the things*
> *I cannot change;*
> *The courage to change the things I can*
> *And the wisdom to know the difference.*

° ° ° O ◯ O ° ° °

Å   *I bless the past with love and let it go. It is easy for me to forgive.*

Å   *I forgive everyone.*

Å   *I forgive myself.*

Where do you want to be physically, personally, financially, professionally and spiritually 6 months from now?

_____

_____

_____

_____

_____

_____

_____

_____

_____

_____

_____

_____

_____

_____

_____

_____

_____

_____

_____

Where do you want to be physically, personally, financially, professionally and spiritually 1 year from now?

_____
_____
_____
_____
_____
_____
_____
_____
_____
_____
_____
_____
_____
_____
_____
_____
_____
_____
_____
_____

*If you always do
What you always did
You'll always be
What you've always been
You'll always get
What you've always got
And you'll always have
What you've always had.*

A successful person is one who builds a firm foundation, not walls, from the bricks thrown at her.

Breathe!

Most of what we see depends upon what we are looking for.

> *Only those who risk going too far
> Can possibly find out how far one can go.*
> — T.S. Eliot

Å *I forgive the past.*

Å *I am free.*

Å *It's easy for me to do what I need to do to take care of myself.*

Å *I am worthy of success.*

Å *I enjoy success in everything I do.*

> *Imagine that there's a zipper at the base of your neck that you can unzip and step out of your fat. Leave it on the chair as, in your imagination, you step out of it. You can mentally communicate with your fat suit and it with you. Your fat suit has something it needs you to know. Listen as your fat suit talks to you. Then you may have something to reply to your fat suit.*
>
> — Nan Bolomey

Å *I always park farther away so I may enjoy walking.*

Å *Nothing tastes as good as thin feels.*

HEALTHY OAT BRAN MUFFINS

2¼ cups oat bran cereal
1 tablespoon baking powder
¼ cup Wax Orchards Fruit Sweet™
1¼ cups nonfat milk
2 very ripe bananas (the riper the better)
2 egg whites
2 tablespoons cold processed canola oil

Add liquid ingredients to dry ingredients. Line muffin tin with paper, fill half full. Bake for 17 minutes at 425° F. Makes about 18 muffins.

Variations: Add 2 to 3 tablespoons Wax Orchard Fudge Sweet™ for "chocolate" muffins. Experiment by adding poppy seeds, almond extract, or other flavorings. Use your imagination.

Five ways that being overweight is working for me:

1 _____
2 _____
3 _____
4 _____
5 _____

What emotions trigger eating for me?

1 _____
2 _____
3 _____
4 _____
5 _____
6 _____
7 _____
8 _____
9 _____

> *For every minute that you are angry*
> *you lose 60 seconds of happiness.*
> — Ralph Waldo Emerson

Learn to say, "What if . . ." instead of "Yes, but . . ."

Seek professional counseling or guidance when needed.

Remember that patience is not just people in a hospital!

> *What other people think of you is none of your business.*
> — Terry Cole-Whittaker

Learn from the past, plan for the future, and live in the present.

Life is 10% what happens to us and 90% how we *choose* to react to it.

Defeat comes from hanging on to solutions that aren't working.

₀ ° o O O O o ° °

There's enough pizza sold in this country *every day* to cover ten Astrodome floors—and it should!

⋯⋯⋯⋯⋯⋯⋯⋯⋯⋯⋯⋯⋯⋯⋯ o ⋯⋯⋯⋯⋯⋯⋯⋯⋯⋯⋯⋯⋯⋯⋯

Buy Rescue Remedy™ in your local health food store. Put 4 drops under your tongue every hour (or whenever you remember). It will reduce your stress and lower resistance to losing weight. No, I don't know how it works but I don't know how aspirin works either. I just know if I ever get a headache, I'll take two and it will go away.

I used to be upset being alone on Friday nights, so I'd eat. Then I realized that on Monday I could pretty well figure Friday would come around in a few days. I started making plans on Monday to do something on Friday!

I used to have a lot of problems. I decided to redefine the word, "problem." I just figured I had lots of situations come up in life that needed to be dealt with. Amazing how few problems I've had in my life from then on!

.... o ....

Keep your bedroom clean and neat. You'll sleep much better.

.... o ....

Drink a glass of warm water with fresh lemon juice in it first thing in the morning. Lemon is a great natural cleanser.

You can do ten pushups in front of the TV in less than 30 seconds. Okay, you can do knee pushups and you don't have to go all the way down. You'll be surprised how quickly you'll build upper body strength just from this.

.... o ....

If you have trouble sleeping at night—and you get up and eat—take .5 mcg of Melatonin at night instead. It's a natural hormone that our bodies stop producing as we age. Take it 20 minutes prior to sleep time.

Å *I easily achieve and maintain my ideal weight.*

Å *I choose what I eat and what I look like.*

Stress produces adrenaline in the body. An overabundance of adrenaline is toxic. Adrenaline is used up by large muscle activity. The largest muscles in your body are your thighs and seat.
To reduce stress, go for a walk.

Twenty minutes is about 1/100th of your day. Walk 10 minutes out and 10 minutes back each day. Walk briskly and swing your arms. You have the time.

Losing weight and getting fit is **not** about looking cute in a bikini! It's about **not** dying and **not** being a vegetable for the last 20 years of your life.

> *Genius is the ability to discern that which is important.*
> *— Albert Einstein*

Breathe!

The only two concepts I want you to consider today are:

- Eat when your body is hungry.

- Do not finish any food today. Leave some of whatever you're eating.

I do this just so that I'll always know **I'm in charge** of what I put into my body. If I eat all the food in front of me, then the food has decided when I stop eating—when its gone!

Prayer for today: "God, help me more."

> *Obstacles are what you see when you take your eyes off your goal.*
> — Hannah More

Å *Today I will practice detachment. I will pretend I am an observer of my life. I will look at the events of my life as lessons and I will focus on what it is I need to learn from them. I will do my best to learn and let go.*

Å *Today I will pay attention to my body's thirst signal. I will drink fresh water as soon as I observe that my body is thirsty.*

Å *I always have enough time, energy, love and money.*

○ ○ ○ ○ ○ ○ ○ ○

When you commit 100% to something, it makes it the easiest thing in the world to do. Because you give yourself no options. When you commit 99% (or less) to something it will drive you crazy because you'll always have that 1% to jerk you around.

When you allow the outer world to dictate your emotions, your life will be like a ping-pong ball in a dryer.

---○---

Å *What I do today will be good enough. I always do the best I can. If I could have done better, I would have done better.*

> *Until one is committed, there is hesitancy, the chance to draw back, always ineffectiveness, concerning all acts of initiative (and creation). There is one elementary truth the ignorance of which kills countless ideas and splendid plans: that the moment one definitely commits oneself, then Providence moves too. All sorts of things occur to help one that would never otherwise have occurred. A whole stream of events issues from the decision, raising in one's favour all manner of unforeseen incidents and meetings and material assistance which no man could have dreamed would have come his way. Whatever you can do or dream you can, begin it. Boldness has genius, power and magic in it. Begin it now.*
>
> — Johann Wolfgang Von Goethe

Read a section of the newspaper you don't normally read. It will encourage your brain to think of other things beside what you normally think of, like food and weight.

- Throw food away—just for practice!

- Practice doing nothing else while you eat but eat.

- Throw away, give away, or put away your bowls. Most of us have bowls that could serve a third world nation—then we have seconds in them! Instead get small ramekins or custard cups. They hold about a fistful.

Å   *I love to eat fresh fruits and vegetables.*

> **COMMITMENT**
> *Commitment is what transforms a promise into reality. It is the words that speak boldly of your intentions and the action which speak louder than words. It is making the time when there is none—coming through time after time, year after year after year. Commitment is the stuff character is made of; the power to change the face of things. It is the daily triumph of integrity over skepticism.*
> — Shearson Lehman
> CEO, American Express

Feel your feelings, don't *eat* them.

○

Conversation about dieting is often a form of denial: We think *talking* about it is the same as *doing* something about it. Listen to how much you discuss food, weight, and the frustrations around both. Then practice stopping yourself from verbally wallowing in it. It will help build energy inside you to actually *do* something about it.

The next time you hear yourself saying (as you're about to put food into your mouth), "Why am I eating? I'm not hungry," *stop* for just a few seconds and let the answer come into your mind. You can always continue eating after you get the answer, however, you may find that you don't want to.

○

Do something *fun* today that doesn't involve food or drink.

Å *Every function in my body is in harmony and balance. I feel better each and every day.*

Make sure your teeth are healthy. It's hard to digest food adequately if it hasn't been chewed properly. If you are a dental/needle phobic, call a hypnotherapist. It usually can be helped fairly easily.

Å *I have a right to a strong, healthy and attractive body. Daily I am more aware.*

Breathe!

When you stay conscious, you open up a world of possibilities. You can choose to eat or not eat **anything at anytime**.

Gauge your hunger on a scale from 1 to 10. One means that your starving—about to pass out from hunger; 10 means that you're stuffed full of food to the point of discomfort. It's the way you feel after Thanksgiving dinner, when you're making that turkey sandwich! Learn your scale and practice eating at a 2 and stopping at a 5. That way you won't get so hungry you'll overeat and when you stop at a 5, your body will use the food you've put into it instead of storing the excess.

1 .... 2 .... 3 .... 4 .... 5 .... 6 .... 7 .... 8 .... 9 10
starving   satisfied   stuffed

Fill in the following spaces with the 5 emotions that come to mind quickest:

I eat when I'm:

_____

_____

_____

_____

_____

Now give yourself some options. Fill in the following blanks with:

Instead of eating when I'm _____,

I could _____.

Instead of eating when I'm _____,

I could _____.

Instead of eating when I'm _____,

I could _____.

Instead of eating when I'm _____,

I could _____.

Instead of eating when I'm _____,

I could _____.

Fill in the following spaces with the names of 5 people who come to mind:

I eat when I'm with:

_____

_____

_____

_____

_____

Now fill in the following spaces:

Instead of eating with _____,

we could _____.

Instead of eating with _____,

we could _____.

Instead of eating with _____,

we could _____.

Instead of eating with _____,

we could _____.

Instead of eating with _____,

we could _____.

BUT WHAT DOES IT MEAN?

An easy guide to food-label terms

You've probably heard talk recently about terms used on food labels. Many new regulations are aimed at helping consumers decide which products are right for their needs. But with all the changing definitions, it can be hard to keep track. Here's a quick guide to the latest FDA/USDA labeling terms.

FREE — Contains no more than the amount that is "nutritionally trivial" and unlikely to have a physiological effect.

FRESH — Can only refer to raw food that hasn't been processed, frozen or preserved.

HIGH — A serving provides 20% or more of the recommended daily intake of the stated nutrient.

LIGHT — Term may be used on foods that have half the fat content of the original product.

MORE — Term may be used to show that a food contains at least 10% more of a desirable nutrient.

SOURCE OF — A serving has 10 to 19% of the recommended daily intake of the nutrient.

SUGAR-FREE — Has less than 0.5 grams of sugar per serving.

CALORIES:

CALORIE FREE — Has less than 5 calories per serving.

LOW CALORIE — Has less than 40 calories per serving and per 100 grams of food.

REDUCED CALORIE — Has 1/3 fewer calories than comparison food.

CHOLESTEROL:

CHOLESTEROL FREE — Has less than 2 milligrams of cholesterol per serving and 2 grams or less of saturated fat per serving.

LOW IN CHOLESTEROL — Has 20 milligrams or less cholesterol per serving and per 100 grams of food, and 2 grams or less of saturated fat.

FAT:

FAT FREE — Has less than 0.5 grams of fat per serving, and no added fat or oil.

LOW FAT — Has 3 grams or less of fat per serving and 100 grams of food.

% FAT FREE — Term may be used only in describing foods that qualify as low fat.

REDUCED FAT — Has no more than 25% the fat of an identified comparison.

LOW IN SATURATED FAT — Has 1 gram or less of saturated fat per serving, and not more than 15% of the calories come from saturated fat.

SALT:

SALT-FREE — Less than 5 milligrams of sodium per serving.

LOW SODIUM — Has less than 140 milligrams of sodium per serving and per 100 grams of food.

VERY LOW SODIUM — Has less than 35 milligrams per serving and per 100 grams of food.

REDUCED SODIUM — Has no more than half the sodium of a comparison food.

Å *I love being a very positive and powerful person.*

When you eat and do anything else like read or watch TV, you have a tendency to go unconscious regarding how much you've eaten. Have you ever looked down in your lap at the empty popcorn bowl and wondered where it all went? Try **just eating** and doing nothing else. You'll be surprised at how quickly you're satisfied and ready to stop eating.

Whenever you say, "I found myself . . ." (i.e., halfway through a doughnut or in front of the ice cream freezer at the supermarket), that assumes you became unconscious for a period of time. Practice making conscious choices throughout your day.

Å *I am accountable for everything I do.*

Å *I am very choosy about the foods I eat. They are always nutritional and satisfying.*

CHICKEN AND RICE

1 cup brown rice
1 can reduced fat cream of mushroom soup <u>or</u> cream of chicken soup
1½ cups water <u>or</u> 1 can nonfat chicken broth
2 chicken breasts, cut up, no skin
1 small can mushrooms with juice

Mix ingredients together and cook on top of the stove at low heat for about 1 hour.

— Julie Tauscher

Often we eat "just to be doing something." Try sitting for 2, 3 or 5 minutes doing nothing. Do the best you can. Become accustomed to allowing your hands to rest in your lap. Practice until you feel comfortable with them at rest.

- Drive by the drive-thru.

- Select an appetizer for your entire dinner at restaurants.

- Split meals at restaurants.

- Remember: Doggie bags were made for thin people.

- Have your server remove the bread or chips from the table **before** you eat any. We often fill up on the bread or chips but order and eat a meal anyway because "that's why we're here."

- At every meal, eat what you like best first. Often we'll "save the best for last" and be full when we get to it and eat it anyway.

- Sit down when you eat.

- Don't eat in the car.

- Clean out your car. Treat yourself to a car wash. See how long you can keep it clean.

- If you haven't worn something for a year, give it away. There's lots of people who can benefit from your "recyclables" and you get the tax deduction!

    I keep an ongoing donation box in a closet. That way, I don't have to decide only once every few months what to give away. I just put it in the box when the mood strikes. I give my donations to a battered women's shelter. I do that with household items too.

Get your life off hold.

If you've been telling yourself "I'll do it when I lose 5, 10, 50 pounds . . . do it ***now***. One of my students had what I thought was gorgeous white hair. She'd been telling herself for years that when she lost 50 pounds, she'd dye her hair auburn. I told her to do it now. She did and immediately began losing weight. It was as if her unconscious said "Hmmm, the hair color changed, I guess I'm losing weight. Okay, I will."

○ ○ ○ ○ ○ ○ ○ ○

When traveling by airplane, find out about the meal options in advance and order a healthy one. They're usually much better than what everyone else gets. If nothing sounds healthy, take your own food onto the plane.

Å *It is a pleasure to live in my body.*

Pay close attention to your self-talk. There are two parts to your brain: the "thinker" and the "prover." The thinker thinks whatever it is you think and the prover sets about to make you right. If you don't want it in your life, stop focusing your attention on it and thereby helping to create it.

> *Argue long enough for your limitations and they are yours.*
> — Richard Bach

Å *I have all the time I need.*

Å *I am always on time easily and effortlessly.*

We can only think one thought at a time. If you find yourself getting upset at what you're thinking, think something else!

Emotions follow thoughts. You may not be able to control what thoughts enter your head, but once they are there, you get to choose whether or not you're going to pay attention to them. This dictates how you feel.

> *Emotions are like waves. Watch them come and go on the vast ocean of existence.*
> — Proverb

If you **must** have chocolate ice cream or whatever it is you think you can't live without at that moment, then by all means have a little bit and be done with it. Because you're going to eat around it until you get to it. And all the celery in the world isn't going to satisfy that chocolate urge.

Å *I choose what I eat and how I look.*
   I joyfully look forward to the future.
   I see only good ahead of me.

When you give yourself permission to eat, tell yourself that you'll have it in an hour. Then go do something else. You may find that if you even think about it in an hour, the urge to eat it will be significantly diminished. Then you may give yourself permission to eat it tomorrow. Or not. See how you expand your range of options when you get out of the knee-jerk habit mode? Isn't this fun?

Å *Every gland, organ and cell in my body is functioning perfectly.*

Å *I love myself and appreciate and respect myself at all times. I am successful in everything I do.*

> **SALMON DIP**
>
> 1 can salmon
> 1 brick no-fat cream cheese
> *to taste:* onion powder
> ....ketchup
> ....salsa
>
> Cream all ingredients together. Great with vegetable sticks or on low-fat crackers.

At restaurants order salad dressing and sauces on the side. Remember, gravy and hollandaise are not ***beverages***. It's what I call the "When Harry Met Sally" mode of ordering. Remember, Sally used to drive everyone crazy the way she was so picky about ordering. Be just like her! I used to own a restaurant. It's a tough business and the only thing that basically distinguishes one restaurant from another is service. Servers know this and will most often do what you ask. If not, I know there's another, better restaurant just down the street that will! I always tell my server, "I know I'm a pain, but I tip well." I always get just what I ask for!

Å *I easily lose weight by changing my eating habits. Because I care about myself, I choose healthy, nutritious and delicious foods.*

Å *I take total responsibility for my life, my body, and the food I eat. I am now totally committed to learning new and healthy ways to express my emotions.*

Don't compare yourself to others. It's a waste of time because you can't walk in their shoes. When we compare, we usually don't fare well in our own minds. Do you really want to feel worse about yourself?

○

You made decisions about the way the world is as a child. What decisions are you still operating on? "Clean your plate" is a common one. Even though your circumstances have changes, the old habit hangs in there. Making conscious choices eliminates old tapes that no longer serve you.

○

Å *I easily say no to foods that are not good for me. I like myself and others like themselves when they are with me. The only reason I eat is for the health and integrity of my body. Losing weight builds a strong, healthy, attractive body. I am a winner.*

> *They can because they think they can.*
> — Virgil

There are two ways to spell waste (waist). What you do with one (the food left on your plate after you've eaten a fistful) will determine the size of the other one!

○

Å *Everything I eat turns to health and beauty.*

You are no longer bound by the confines of "breakfast" or "lunch" or "dinner" food. If you want soup for breakfast, by all means have it! Expand your thinking!

○

If you don't volunteer, try it. If you volunteer too much, begin saying "no." Say it several times out loud when you're alone, just for practice!

○

Eat **nothing** from its original container, especially ice cream, Chinese take-out, chips, and microwave popcorn.

PROTEIN ENERGY BARS

1 cup Spiru-tein powder (At health food stores.
   I use vanilla; chocolate is good, too.)
1 cup rolled oats
1 cup whole wheat flour
¼ cup bran
2 small boxes raisins
¼ cup sunflower seeds
¼ cup orange or apple frozen concentrate
¼ cup fruit sweetener (at health food stores)
3 egg whites, with 1 tablespoon vanilla added

Mix all together and pat into a 9" x 11" cooking sheet or flat pan sprayed lightly with a nonstick coating. If mixture is too dry, add additional liquid, such as water or more fruit concentrate. Bake in 350° F. oven for 20 minutes or until lightly brown.

— Julie Tauscher

When ordering Chinese food, say "No MSG, please," and order nothing deep-fried or sweet and sour. Order one dish for every two people. Have leftovers boxed up immediately, so you don't sit there and pick after you've eaten a fistful.

When eating at a Mexican restaurant, say, "Please take the chips away and bring me a tortilla instead." (They're steamed, not deep-fried.) Order nothing fried and **no** cheese on anything. You'll be amazed how good the food actually tastes when it's not covered with cheese—which makes it taste all the same.

Throw away the deep fryer. The oil and heat kill nutrition in your food.

- Sauté food in fat-free broth or water or Pam™.

Pork is **not** the "other white meat." It's usually the fattiest meat you can buy.

GREAT QUICK HEALTHY DINNER FOR ONE

In a small amount of water, boil a peeled, quartered potato with ½ a quartered onion until nearly tender.

Add a piece of fresh fish (I like a small piece of Chilean sea bass) for about 5 minutes or until it flakes apart. Great fish stew!

Å *I love my hands. My nails are long and strong. My cuticles are smooth and healthy.*

Imagine yourself standing on a scale and looking down and seeing the number you want there.

·······o·······

When cooking hamburger for spaghetti, buy it lean and rinse it in a colander after cooking. This gets the excess grease off of it.

·······o·······

Stop making excuses.

> *Whatever you are ready for*
> *is ready for you.*
> — Reverend Ike

Some of you may be familiar with the following saying; however, many of you may not know it in its entirety:

> *When the student is ready, the teacher will appear . . . everywhere.*

·······o·······

Å ***I spend time each day in creative pursuits.***

Å ***I spend time each day increasing my general and/or professional knowledge.***

Å ***I spend time each week cultivating new and old friendships and enjoy the time.***

Make a list of five answers to the following question:

What do I need to complete in my life?

1. _____
2. _____
3. _____
4. _____
5. _____

Do one of them a week.

₀ ° ο Ο Ο Ο ο ° °

If you ever get sick and lose your appetite, don't "force yourself to eat."

- If you ever get a sore throat, try rubbing a little Neosporin® on the outside of your throat.

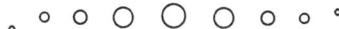

Make your bed in the morning. It's a small way to begin to feel better about yourself. When you feel better about yourself, losing weight is easier.

> Prayer for today:
> *"God give me the strength to do what I have to do today and the grace to do it well."*
> — Joel Junker

If you have a task to do that seems daunting (cleaning out a desk or closet, for example), set the timer for 10 minutes and just work on that task for that amount of time. Do it every day. It'll be completed before you know it! Often we don't start projects because they seem just too big. Break them down into manageable parts. The same with weight loss. It's a day at a time or an hour at a time. Sometimes it's a minute at a time.

> *Our greatest glory is not in never falling,*
> *But in rising every time we fall.*
> — Confucius

I subscribe to "Inspire." Each morning on my e-mail I find a saying or story which is inspirational. I encourage anyone with e-mail to subscribe. It's free. The address on the Internet is: **http://www.infoadvn.com/inspire/**

I also subscribe to "Success Online" which periodically e-mails me exactly what I need to motivate me that day. The e-mail address is: patlav@epix.net. It's also free.

Å **Every day is fun for me. I enjoy all of my life.**

Å **I love to learn new things. Learning is easy for me.**

Å **I always have enough time, energy, love, and money.**

> *Kindness is within our power even when fondness is not.*
> — Samuel Johnson

When my husband Walter died, I immediately lost 15 pounds. The following month I gained nearly 30 pounds Do you know how much food you have to eat to gain a pound a day? *A lot!* There was no place for me to go and talk. Any support groups for widowed people were for older people. I was in my mid-30s.

A few years ago I met Joel Junker, who had lost his young wife to cancer six months before Walter died. Together, with others in the same boat, we began WYPS—Widowed Young Person's Support. It's been helping people get through their pain since 1991. In our spare time, Joel, Kath McCormack, Barbara Thrasher-Meyers, and I travel around the country helping communities set up WYPS. If you know anyone who has recently lost a spouse and is young, have them call me at 1-888-763-5444 to find the group nearest them or to get support in creating one.

If you are grieving a loss, get the book, *How to Survive the Loss of A Love,* by Peter McWilliams.

Every loss you have experienced needs to be grieved. Fill the hole in your soul with nurturing instead of pizza.

₀ ∘ ○ ◯ ◯ ○ ∘ °

Å ***I am a beloved child of God, protected by Divine Love and Light at all times.***

Do one thing today that you've been putting off. Take note of how quickly it got accomplished compared to how much brain time was spent on procrastinating. Let your new motto be:
"When it comes up I handle it."

DEEP AT THE CENTER OF MY BEING

There is an infinite well of love. I now allow this love to flow to the surface. It fills my heart, my body, my mind, my consciousness, my very being and radiates out from me in all directions and returns to me multiplied. The more love I use and give, the more I have to give; the supply is endless. The use of love makes me feel good. It is an expression of my inner joy.

I love myself

Therefore I take loving care of my body. I lovingly feed it nourishing food and beverages. I lovingly groom and dress it. And my body lovingly responds to me with vibrant health and energy.

I love myself

Therefore, I provide for myself a comfortable home, one that fills all of my needs and is a pleasure to be in. I fill the rooms with the vibration of love so that all who enter, myself included, will feel this love and be nourished by it.

I love myself

Therefore, I work at a job that I truly enjoy doing, one that uses my creative talents and abilities, working with and for people who I love and who love me and earning a good income.

I love myself

Therefore I behave and think in a loving way to all people for I know that that which I give out returns to me multiplied. I only attract loving people in my world for they are a mirror or myself.

I love myself

Therefore I forgive and totally release the past and all past experiences. I am free.

I love myself

Therefore I love totally in the now, experiencing each moment as good and knowing that my future is bright, joyous and secure for I am a beloved child of the Universe and the Universe lovingly takes care of me now and forever more.

(Author unknown)

Learn something new today. It'll start to get you out of only dwelling on "food, weight, dieting, etc."

Estimates suggest that 78% of Americans are sleep-deprived. When you're tired you may think you need to eat more to "keep up your strength." Digesting food is one of the most energy-depleting activities our bodies do.

Sleeping in a cooler, rather than warmer room facilitates better sleep.

Do **not** use an electric blanket. Use a comforter. You'll sleep better and burn calories keeping warm as you sleep.

If you have a stressful job, you need a peaceful home life. If you have a stressful home life, you need a peaceful job. When you create some peace in your life, you'll have fewer problems to eat about.

Men, to facilitate a peaceful home life with your partner, don't ever give her a gift that plugs in, unless she specifically requests it. Remember a vacuum cleaner is the gift that keeps on sucking!

To facilitate a peaceful home life, opposite sexes generally shouldn't go to the mall together. You see, men go shopping. Women go **shopping**. That's usually a setup for conflict!

> **CHANGE**
> *Everybody thinks of changing humanity*
> *and nobody thinks of changing himself.*
> — Leo Tolstoy

Ten ways I could let others love me are:

1. _____
2. _____
3. _____
4. _____
5. _____
6. _____
7. _____
8. _____
9. _____
10. _____

I want to lose weight because:

_____
_____
_____
_____
_____
_____
_____

My ideal vacation would be:

_____
_____
_____
_____
_____

My ideal career would be:

_____
_____
_____
_____
_____

Today I was inspired by:

_____
_____
_____
_____
_____
_____

Å *I feel good about myself because everything I put in my mouth is good for me. I wouldn't put it in my mouth if it wasn't.*

GINGER DRESSING

1 can no-fat chicken broth
¼ cup balsamic vinegar
¼ cup rice vinegar
1 or 2 tablespoons of grated ginger
3 cloves of garlic finely chopped
few drops of sesame oil for flavor
few flakes of red pepper

If the flavor is too strong, add a little water. Let it sit overnight to blend. Use as marinade or dressing.

— Julie Tauscher

Å *Today I will eat slower, enjoying and savoring each bite of food. I will stay present and conscious and as soon as my body tells me it has had enough food, I will stop eating regardless of where I am, how much the food cost, who I am with or what the food is. I know that I have access to any food I could possibly want any time of the day or night. It's not necessary to eat it all right now.*

Å *My arms are long, slender, and firm. My legs are strong, long, and lean. My stomach is flat.*

Å *I become more beautiful every day. I love the way I look.*

People who irritate you:

Although there are many reasons for interpersonal conflict, I've found the following three to be among the most common:

1. People with whom you have "unfinished business"—that is, there's something you need to clear the air about but haven't had the courage or the time "just wasn't right" to confront, or

2. People who *remind* you of someone with whom you have unfinished business, or

3. People who reflect back to you your own "stuff." After all, it's so much easier to see it in someone else than in ourselves! In any case, each scenario offers you the opportunity to "eat your words."

Exercises to heal people-irritants in your life:

▶ *Be in a quiet room where you won't be disturbed for about 10 minutes. Place two chairs about 3 feet apart, facing each other. Sit in one and imagine the person who irritates you in the other chair. Tell him/her exactly how you feel. You can be angry, sad, matter-of-fact—just be however you feel. Be as brief or as long as you like. Then sit in the other chair as though you were that person and respond to yourself. You may be amazed at what comes out of your mouth. Keep switching chairs until you feel a sense of completion.*

You'll feel much lighter at the end of this exercise. A word of caution: On some level, the other person may perceive a reduction in your hostility (oh, yes, despite your attempts to show that everything's alright, they **do** perceive that it's not!) and may call you out of the blue. Or you may be surprised at how much nicer that person is the next time you see him/her. It's a great opportunity to heal relationships. By the way, it doesn't matter if the other person is dead or alive. Death doesn't heal old wounds. This exercise does. If you were seriously abused by this person, I recommend counseling before attempting this exercise.

For the perfectionists who delay this exercise until you get the verbiage exactly right–do it now! It doesn't have to be perfect. You can always do it again when you remember more. Besides, intention is a great part of it. Just putting the chairs together begins the healing process.

▶ **Look hard at what it is that irritates you about other people. Pinpoint it and then look within yourself—not judgmentally, but dispassionately, as an observer.**

Remember, an oyster makes a priceless pearl from a grain of sand through *irritation!* Often those who irritate us the most are our greatest teachers.

If you are a jealous person, for example, you may attract to you people who will afford you the opportunity to be jealous. *They* don't make you jealous. You attracted them into your life so you can be who you already are! If you keep attracting people who can't commit, **maybe** there's something about you that is afraid of commitment. There's a tendency in this country to blame men for commitment-phobia. It's entirely possible that we're placing the blame on the wrong gender. At least let's look at our own accountability.

> *When you are offended at any man's fault, turn to yourself and study your own failings. Then you will forget your anger.*
> — Epicetetus

Å *I have abundant recreation, acceptance, attention, and social interaction without eating.*

Exert your will today. Do one thing that's best for you just to practice being in charge of your life.

When you slow down, time slows down with you. What that means is when you take the time to think something through and do it right the first time, you'll save a lot of time and energy ***not*** redoing it.

Make something today. One theory of obesity states that when a person's creativity is stifled, overeating occurs. Make a friend, make a bouquet, make a quilt—make something!

Today, remember something from your childhood that brought you joy.

Today, expect guidance from the unexpected.

₀ ∘ o O ◯ O o ∘ °

Å   *I accept myself. I accept my body. I love my body.*

Å   *I love my body more every day. My body is healthy, fit, and strong. My body is beautiful.*

This is one of my favorite writings. It helps make our basic fear of death less fearful:

THE LEGACY

When I die, give what is left of me to children.
If you need to cry, cry for your brothers and sisters
  walking beside you.
Put your arms around anyone and give them
  what you need to give to me.
I want to leave you with something, something
  better than words or sounds.
Look for me in the people I have known and loved.
And if you cannot live without me, then let me
  live on in your eyes, your mind and your acts
  of kindness.
You can love me most by letting hands touch
  hands and letting go of children that need
  to be free.
Love does not die, people do.
So when all that is left of me is love . . .
Give me away.

(author unknown)

Å *I am filled with joy and happiness. There is so much happiness in my life. I awaken each morning fresh, alert, energetic, and happy. I begin and end each day with a smile. I am full of praise and gratitude.*

The 5 most inspirational people in my life are:

1. _____
2. _____
3. _____
4. _____
5. _____

They inspire me because:

1. _____
2. _____
3. _____
4. _____
5. _____

ICE CREAM SANDWICH

2 plain cookie biscuits (such as Petite Beurre™ with 1 gram of fat per cookie)
¼ cup no fat, no sugar added ice cream (Dreyer's® is best)
1 teaspoon all fruit jelly, any flavor

Make an ice cream sandwich between the two biscuits. No deprivation here!

— Julie Tauscher

Today be a little selfish. You can only take care of others to the extent that you can take care of yourself.

You can only love others to the extent that you can show yourself love.

○

Your Spirit is incredibly powerful. It needs a healthy body to begin to demonstrate its power.

○

There are those who would tell you that first you must love your body. Then you can lose weight. I'm not one of the people who would tell you that. I know a lot of skinny people who hate their bodies. What I will ask you to do is respect your body. Because, let's face it, for all the abuse we've heaped on them, for the most part, they're still carrying us around! When you begin to respect your body, you'll **want** to put fewer toxins in it. And when you do that, your body will respond by feeling better. Then you may begin to like each other a little more. Love may or may not come later. It probably will.

> *... the healthy, the strong individual, is the one who asks for help when s/he needs it whether s/he's got an abscess on the knee or in the soul.*
> — Rona Barrett

Å *Today will be my teacher and my mirror.*

Å *Today has opportunities to succumb to the wishes of others. Today I will take the time to assess my own feelings rather than say "yes" out of fear that they won't like me if I say "no."*

Å *I choose what I eat and how I look.*

Å *My Spirit is strong and powerful and only operates for my own good. I trust where it will take me.*

> *In nature there are neither rewards or punishments—only consequences.*
> — Robert G. Ingersoll

Å *I am wonderfully worthy of giving and receiving unconditional love.*

Å *I am always on time and love the feeling of being on time.*

Å *I am very choosy about the foods I eat. They are always nutritional and satisfying.*

Å *I am blessed with good, dedicated, and exciting friends.*

> *Any idea seriously entertained tends to bring about the realization of itself.*
> — Joseph Chilton Pearce

Å *I easily earn and enjoy earning $_____ a year. I have $_____ in my savings account at all times. I am effortlessly free from debt.*

You have a contract with everyone in your life; this contract is unwritten and unspoken. But it is a powerful basis for **why** you are in each other's lives. Oftentimes your weight is part of the contract, and when you begin to lose weight, you are *unilaterally and arbitrarily* changing the contract. If, for example, a partner is insecure, as we all are in varying degrees, s/he may offer you food to "reward" you for doing so well on your diet. This is sabotage. Politely, say, "No, thank you." Be aware that they probably *don't even know what they're doing!* It's a perfect opportunity to practice communicating and asking for what you want and updating your contracts.

> *Our greatest happiness does not depend on the condition of life in which chance has placed us, but is always the result of a good conscience, good health, occupation and freedom in all just pursuits.*
> — Thomas Jefferson

Remember, the **only** thing you can control is yourself. Today practice releasing the need to control the people and events in your life. You may be surprised at how exquisitely life resolves itself *without* your help. This leads to fewer disappointments in life and thus, fewer reasons to eat.

---------- o ----------

Å *I respond more and more to the energy and joy I am obtaining. There is within me enough time, energy and money to accomplish everything I desire. My days are filled with pleasures as I give out love and receive love. My consciousness is expanding.*

Å *Every day and in every way I am growing younger, stronger and more prosperous. I am a very positive person.*

POTATO TOPPING OR DIP

1 ounce of Uncle Dan's or Hidden Valley Dressing™
½ cup thick and chunky salsa
1 pint no-fat sour cream

Mix together and blend overnight.

— Julie Tauscher

Two monks in ancient Japan were walking along and spied a bride on her way to her wedding. They were standing next to a river and the bride appeared distressed at being unable to cross the river without getting wet and muddy. One of the monks offered to carry her across the river. Gratefully, she climbed up on his shoulders and they crossed the river. The monk deposited her on the opposite side of the river, she thanked him and they went their separate ways.

About a mile down their path, the monk who did not carry the woman turned to the other monk and said in a rage, "I can't believe you did that!"

*Puzzled, the first monk asked to what was he referring. The monk replied, "You **touched** a woman! You know it is forbidden to **touch a woman**."*

*Whereupon the first monk gently replied "Ah, yes, brother, in aiding the woman it was necessary to touch her. But **I** put her down a mile back."*

> *What is this life if, full of care,*
> *We have no time to stand and stare?*
> — William Henry Davies

In 1987, a survey was taken of CEOs of Fortune 500 companies. The results were surprising. A large response to the survey was received—over 8% (the norm is 1 to 3%). It was discovered that a vast majority of the respondents felt that they really weren't as good as others around them thought they were; that they were "pulling the wool" over the eyes of their peers and subordinates and that if they were ever "found out," they would lose their titles, positions, and responsibilities.

Sound like anyone you know?

In 1988, a study was conducted at the University of Pittsburgh. In this study, lab mice were put on diets for a period of time, then allowed to eat as they wished, then put back on the diet, then taken off. This was repeated several times and the results showed that each time they were put on the diet, they lost less weight and each time the restrictions were removed they gained more.

Anybody surprised?

> *When we cling to pain we end up punishing ourselves.*
> — Leo Buscaglia

Å ***Everything I eat turns into a strong and healthy body. I do not reach for food to eat when I am not hungry.***

Your parents may have spoken critically or harshly to you as a child, but they can't hold a candle to how badly you talk to yourself. When you find yourself putting you down, **stop it**. You are in charge of your life. Take control of the language you use with yourself and it may help you treat you kinder.

> *No one can make you feel inferior without your consent.*
> *— Eleanor Roosevelt*

Your excess weight comes to you bearing many gifts—one of which is a doorway to your soul. When you choose to accept the gifts, the messenger (your weight) can leave.

> *The change of one simple behavior can affect other behaviors and thus change many things.*
> *— Jean Baer*

Your body won't lie to you. Your brain will jerk you around seven ways from Sunday! But your body will let you know when it wants food and when to stop eating. *Listen to it*. Learn to differentiate between your body's signals and your brain playing with you.

Å   *There is a wide range of foods I eliminate from my world. My body rejects bad foods. They do not smell good. I eliminate sugar in all forms. I do not eat sugar. I have no desire for sugar. I have no desire for caffeine.*

What if you bet on yourself—and didn't lose?

My 10 greatest pleasures are:

1 _____
2 _____
3 _____
4 _____
5 _____
6 _____
7 _____
8 _____
9 _____
10 _____

Ten ways I could love myself are:

1 _____
2 _____
3 _____
4 _____
5 _____
6 _____
7 _____
8 _____
9 _____
10 _____

> *I have found that most people are about as happy as they make up their minds to be.*
> — Abraham Lincoln

> *If you find your inner conversation running along negative lines, you have the power to change the subject, to think along different lines.*
> — Martha Smock

Pain is inevitable.
Suffering is optional.

> *Good people are good*
> *Because they've come to wisdom*
> *Through failure*
> — William Saroyan

Consider the possibility that you've never failed. Yes, including your weight loss efforts. You may have tried many things and if they didn't give you the result you wanted, you stopped doing them and looked for other things that would work better. I'd call that success! And if you learned something along the way, Great Success!

> *A hard beginning makes a good ending.*
> — John Heywood

Rewrite some of your history today. Your past is what you believe it to be. Change your mind about something today.

Å **I easily separate all emotions from hunger, and I only eat when my body is hungry.**

What do you long for?

_____
_____
_____
_____
_____
_____
_____
_____

What can/will you do to create it?

_____
_____
_____
_____
_____
_____
_____
_____
_____

> *Not being beautiful was the true blessing*
> *Not being beautiful forced me to develop*
> *My inner resources*
> *The pretty girl has a handicap to overcome.*
> — Golda Meir

In your spare time today, imagine yourself with your ideal body. Imagine how you would act to maintain this body. Feel this slender, lean body. Notice how happy you are, how much energy you have, how light you feel.

> *To oppose something*
> *Is to maintain it.*
> — Ursula K. LeGuin

Give yourself permission to eat what you want. Notice I didn't say *eat* whatever you want! Just give yourself permission to do so. Because right now, you're putting up all these arbitrary rules about your food and eating behavior and *it's not working!* When you give yourself permission, you take the power away from the food and give it to your body. You see, if you continually deny yourself a hamburger, it has to get bigger and bigger to beat you. It could turn into three burgers before it wins. And when you give yourself permission to eat, then you can also give yourself permission *not to eat.*

> *We win half the battle*
> *When we make up our minds*
> *To take the world as we find it,*
> *Including the thorns.*
> — Orison S. Marden

> *Happiness depends, as Nature shows,*
> *less on exterior things than most suppose.*
> — William Cowper

If there was a part of you that thinks you need to be overweight, what would the name of that part be?

> *The weakest among us has a gift,*
> *however seemingly trivial,*
> *which is peculiar to him*
> *and which worthily used*
> *will be a gift also to his race.*
> — John Ruskin

Give someone the benefit of the doubt today. **Lighten Up!**

> *Without courage,*
> *All other virtues*
> *Lose their meaning.*
> — Sir Winston Churchill

Today eat only when you're hungry.

Notice how often you play the "When/Then" Myth. It goes something like this: *When* I lose this weight, *then* I will _____ (you fill in the blank). The problem with this myth is it keeps you in the future and out of the present and change can only occur in the present. Let me help you out. **When** you lose weight **then** you will have a smaller body. That's it. The rest of your life will be up to you as it always has been.

QUIZ

What is your weight taking the blame for that it doesn't deserve the blame for?

_____

_____

_____

_____

_____

_____

_____

_____

How is being overweight keeping you safe?

_____

_____

_____

_____

_____

_____

_____

_____

Å *I love being a nonsmoker. I feel proud and powerful being a nonsmoker.*

Å *Every morning at 6:00 a.m, I enjoy walking on my treadmill. That time always provides a much appreciated time for reaffirming my goals and planning my day.*

Å *I only spend what I can afford to spend.*

Å *I now deal confidently with being a sexually attractive person, and I love being attractive.*

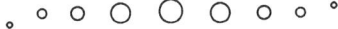

Five votes of confidence:

1. Today I refuse to be shackled by yesterday's memories.

2. Today what I don't know will no longer intimidate me. I will instead view it as an opportunity.

3. Today I will not allow others to define my mood, my method, my image or my mission.

4. Today I will pursue a mission greater than myself by making at least one person happy that s/he saw me.

5. Today I will not tolerate self-pity, gossip or negativism—from myself or others.

STUFFED MUNCHKIN PUMPKINS

1 handful of wild rice, soaked in water for a day or overnight
2 handfuls of basmati or jasmine rice
1 handful of coarsely chopped walnuts or pumpkin seeds
2 handfuls of coarsely chopped mushrooms (chanterelles are perfect)
2 handfuls of dried cranberries
4 miniature pumpkins (remove seeds from pumpkin and top and save)
2 tablespoons olive oil (optional)
¼ teaspoon sage
¼ teaspoon rosemary
⅛ teaspoon curry powder
½ teaspoon salt
½ teaspoon pepper

After soaking wild rice for 8 to 12 hours, bring the water to boil and add white rice. Cook, covered, on low heat until white rice is cooked but firm. If necessary, add a little water before it is done to prevent burning.

Add the remaining ingredients. Stir while cooking until all ingredients are hot and moistened. Water should be cooked off at this point. Stuff the pumpkins or refrigerate the rice mixture for use within the next two days.

After stuffing, put the pumpkin tops on top of rice and place on lightly oiled roasting pan. Bake, covered, in a 350º F oven for 45 to 60 minutes.

You always do the best you can. If you could have done better, you would have done better.
— Katie Evans

FOR A "SAFE AND SANE" THANKSGIVING HOLIDAY

(as far as eating and stress go!)

Although many of you may be accustomed to feeling like the martyr during the holidays, most of the rest of us find it quite a bore. So LIGHTEN UP! on yourself and others! Here's some ideas on how to do just that:

- If you're having guests for dinner on Thanksgiving, meet them at the door with a decoratively trimmed basket containing slips of paper upon which you've written all the little things that need to be done before and after the meal. This could be setting the table, preparing appetizers, clearing the table, doing dishes, putting leftovers away. Have each guest pick a slip and thereby becoming a participant in creating the festivities and allowing you to enjoy the holiday.

- If you're having people bring a dish for dinner, suggest that they "low-fat" a favorite. Bet no one will even know and don't tell anyone! If you're a guest, do the same.

- When preparing mashed potatoes, use the water from boiling the potatoes instead of milk and butter. It's where the nutrients are and again, no one will even notice. Roast coarsely chopped garlic to sprinkle on top of potatoes to give it crunch and flavor.

- Send each of your guests home with a doggy bag. That will get most of the food out of your house so you won't be tempted to eat all weekend.

- If you use prepared stuffing mix, omit the butter or margarine. Again, no one will know the difference-except your waistline.

- If you use turkey drippings to make gravy, first pour it into a jar and put into the freezer for about half an hour. This makes it easy to pull off the layer of fat from the top.

- Take a brisk walk the morning of any holiday. This starts the day off with lots of energy and you won't feel as guilty if you overeat. Walk or bike to your holiday gathering if possible. Get a map and involve the whole family in the adventure of choosing a route.

- Create new traditions. Reassess the way you spend your time on the holidays. If you're tired of watching "Uncle Joe" pass out after dinner, plan to spend your day somewhere else.

- Remember, our Thanksgiving holiday is just that—a day to be thankful for our many blessings. If our forefathers had wanted it to be "Eat Until You Explode and Wish You Were Dead Day" they would have named it that! Make moderation, relaxation and joy your words for the day. God Bless.

○ ○ ○ ○ ○ ○ ○ ○

Å *This week I am losing ___ pounds.*

Å *This month I am losing ___ pounds.*

Å *My metabolism now processes all food to maintain my ideal weight of ___ pounds.*

Å *These affirmations are true for me.*

FOCUS:

F—ollow
O—ne
C—ourse
U—ntil
S—uccessful

Whatever you focus your attention on is what will show up in your life. Focus on what you want.

When you say to yourself, for example, "I won't eat that last piece of pie in the kitchen", your brain goes to the object of the sentence—"pie". **Then** it goes to what activity you want to happen about that object—"won't eat." However, it usually gets stuck on the object. That's why you generally say to yourself, "Oh, what the heck. I'll just eat it then it will be gone, then I won't have to think about it any more."

- In a recent study, it was found that the number one predictor of who would receive a promotion in a bank was the people who *dressed* like management. What we can learn from this is to *act as if you already had whatever it is to which you aspire*. Now, this doesn't mean spend money before you have it. It means to feel and act and look as if you have it—whether it's a new healthy body or a promotion or whatever your heart desires.

- According to Napoleon Hill, author of *Think and Grow Rich*, there are two parts to the brain: the transmitter and the receiver. Whatever frequency you're transmitting on is the one you will receive on. It's an inside job! If you don't like what's going on in the world around you, change what's going on within you.

Have fun playing with your brain and creating the life you want today.

> **Beginning**
> *He who is outside the door*
> *has already a good part*
> *of his journey behind him*
> — Dutch Proverb

Begin immediately visualizing, imagining, and feeling your ideal body. Do not look in the mirror and criticize.

You have a picture of the way the world is in your mind. It matters little if that is the way the world really is—your perception is your truth. Therefore, if you "see" yourself in your mind's eye as overweight—that's your truth. Remember one of the primary functions of the brain is to maintain your sanity. I don't believe you can work against one of the primary brain jobs. You need to learn to work with it!

When you go on a diet and your body gets smaller and you haven't changed the picture in your brain, *the difference between the body in the mirror and picture or image of the body in your brain could make you crazy!* Remember, the picture in your brain is the **truth.** This discrepancy could be responsible in part for the weight you regain after the latest diet. *Your body will move toward the picture that you hold in your mind.*

Change the image of your body that you have in your mind today.

> **Action**
> *To do anything in this world worth doing,*
> *We must not stand back shivering*
> *And thinking of the cold and danger,*
> *but jump in and scramble through*
> *As well as we can.*
> — Sydney Smith

What makes you happy?

_____
_____
_____
_____
_____
_____
_____

What makes you sad?

_____
_____
_____
_____
_____
_____
_____

Women generally will overestimate the size of their bodies. That is, they'll look in the mirror and see a body that's larger than it really is. Men tend to do the opposite.

Another benefit to changing your body in your mind, while your changing it in the mirror, is that since the picture in your mind is the truth, you will begin to eat to support the weight of the body in your brain.

Listen to your self-talk. Eliminate phrases like "I'm a fat pig" from your vocabulary *now*. If you don't want to **be** it, don't *say* it.

Results occur when behavior changes.

If you want to know who someone **is**, watch what s/he **does**.

The unconscious mind has no logic and no rationale. It operates on emotions. The predominant emotion in the unconscious is fear, specifically fear of change. Another reason dieting doesn't work is that often it's a radical behavior change which brings up fear. This can trigger the defenses of the subconscious to kick in and cause you to sabotage yourself sooner or later. To avoid this, lose weight slowly and gradually keeping an open dialogue with the unconscious regarding the emotions you are feeling and just allow yourself to feel them and work through them. You may need the help of a counselor or therapist. I recommend hypnotherapy.

. ° ○ ○ ◯ ○ ○ ° .

Å *I often listen to self-improvement tapes. Every time I listen to them, I enter deep Alpha level with full awareness and complete control.*

Meditation to Get Off Junk Food:

*Think of the most disgusting thing you can imagine. Really get into it. See it, smell it, taste it, feel it. Use all of your senses to make it real for you. (When I first tried this for myself I had decided I wanted to eliminate diet pop. I imagined a big hairy spider leg coming **out of** the pop can). Put that in the back of your mind. Now imagine the food or beverage your want gone from your life (if it's too scary to imagine it gone forever, just assume it's just gonna be gone for awhile; you can always bring it back). Imagine that you are about to take a bite or drink of it and right before it gets to your mouth bring the disgusting image to the front of your mind. Focus all of your attention on the gross image.*

Do this 3 times and you simply won't think of that eliminated food again. Your brain won't let you. Of course, as I mentioned you can always override this self-programming. But why would you want to?

A powerful motivating force of the subconscious is to avoid embarrassment. This is often why we don't try new activities. We're afraid we'll be embarrassed. A little tip: most people are far too interested in how they look to worry about how you look! Try something new today.

Safety
Prudence which degenerates into timidity
Is very seldom the path to safety.
— Viscount Cecil

Fear of change is a common, universal fear. Ironically, the only guarantee we have is that things will change. Acceptance of this one simple fact will make your life significantly easier.

I used to be a "closet eater"—
I'd eat closets full of food at one time!

I used to think "grazing" was an Olympic event. I'd get my Reeboks™ on and start at one end of the kitchen and go through the cupboards and fridge, just to see what "looked good". A little tip from me to you: If you're looking for what *looks* good, you're **not hungry**. Chances are you're either bored or using food to procrastinate. It's a perfect opportunity to **stop** and ask yourself, "What am I really feeling?" You can always still choose to eat. However, injecting a little rationale into the middle of an emotional experience is a powerful start to being in charge of your life (the goal of this program).

THOUGHTS
Watch your thoughts; they become words.
Watch your words; they become actions.
Watch your actions; they become habits.
Watch your habits; they become character.
Watch your character; for it becomes your destiny.
— Author unknown

Watch your "all or nothing" thinking. Begin to discover all the shades of the rainbow called life—between the black and white thinking that we often do. As one of my students so wisely put it, "If you've only come up with two answers, you haven't begun to solve the problem."

--------------------------------- o ---------------------------------

Å *I enjoy life.*
I end each day with gratitude.
I sleep peacefully.
All is well in my world.

Most humans (especially overweight ones) are what we call "externally referenced." That is, if we *see* or *hear about* a food, it could trigger the desire to *eat* that food. Where we're going is to be "internally referenced." That means "If I'm hungry and my body is asking for that food, I'll eat it." *Regardless* of where we are, what food is in front of us, who paid for it or who we're with. Now, **that's** being in charge of your life!

If you have children, **don't** teach them how to eat. They already know. What you are actually teaching them is your bad habits about eating. Are you sure you want to pass that on? The only restrictions I would put on a child's eating is to minimize sugar products. I call "goodies" "baddies." Making a child eat foods they don't like or eating when they're not hungry ("just one more bite") is "food abuse." Don't do it. Did you like it when it was done to you? Did it help you create the relationship with food you want? No. Your kids will be healthier and have fewer food issues if you don't pass yours on to them. Tell your relatives to leave the kids alone about food, too. Understand they mean well but it's usually not in the best interest of the child.

Many people eat when they're tired to "keep up their strength." When you're tired, take a couple of minutes to completely relax your body while saying to yourself, "When I open my eyes in two minutes, I will have had a 20-minute nap." With a little practice, you'll be amazed at how well this will re-energize you. And there's one more thing you don't have to "eat about."

Sometimes people say to me, "If I learn to love my body the way it is, I'm afraid it won't change." To which I respond, "Hey, you don't love it the way it is and it's *not* changing now. Let's just try something different."

"Consider the possibility."

Many people believe that hypnotherapists make you unconscious. Actually, quite the opposite is true. Most of our lives are lived unconsciously. What a good hypnotherapist will strive to do is help you find brief moments of consciousness and focus so that you know how they feel. You can use these moments to decide who you want running your life (you or that Twinkie) and you become more comfortable staying conscious and present.

A study was done several years ago which hypothesized that if science could build a computer that could do everything one human brain could do, that computer would be the size of Texas and three stories high. I have a friend, Robin, who's a computer "techie." He figures that given the new advances in computers, the size may only be the state of Washington now. It's still pretty mind-boggling!

Å *I enjoy relaxing with my weight management tapes each day. The depth of relaxation reached with my tapes increases daily.*

Å *I truly believe in the power of my affirmations.*

SUGGESTIONS FOR HALLOWEEN AND THE HOLIDAYS BEYOND:

1. If you're going to have trick-or-treaters at your house, buy candy for them that you don't like! This will keep you out of it while waiting to give it away.

2. Better yet, buy apples, stickers, pogs, or toothbrushes (available *cheap* from a dental supply house) for trick-or-treaters.

3. After two days, put all leftover candy in plastic bags and place in the back of your freezer where you'll forget about it until it's freezer burned, or

4. Take all leftover candy to work—or just throw it away!

5. Remember that remnants of rat hair, teeth, and feces have been found in packaged candy. Bon appetit!

6. Use your imagination and create a costume from clothing available at second-hand stores such as Goodwill. You'll save money and support a worthy cause at the same time.

7. If you're planning on taking goodies to your child's school Halloween party, choose something healthy like apples, pears or grapes. If you're baking, use Wax Orchards Fruit Sweet® instead of sugar.

8. Find a low-fat recipe for pumpkin bread and bake it as cupcakes.

9. If you have a "sweet tooth," try taking 200 mcg. of chromium picolinate. Follow the recommended dosage; it should cut sugar cravings. If you have a tendency to snack on sweets at night, take it between 4:00 and 6:00 p.m.

10. To cut down on stress during the next few months, listen to a meditation tape prior to going to sleep at night. You'll sleep deeper and get more rest in the same amount of time.

11. If you have small children, create a "Babysitter Exchange" with your neighbors who also have children. Use it for a needed parental break as well as to get shopping done.

12. DELEGATE. Ask for help when you need it!

Overweight people often tell me that they feel that food and eating are the only aspect of their lives over which they have control. What's wrong with that sentence? Eating until you can't move is *not* being in control. What they often really mean is that it's the only time they think they can do what they want. A quick way to fix that situation is to take back control in other areas of life. In other words, bring more balance into life. More control in all areas of your life means less need to "just do what I want" because you're doing what you want more often overall.

The opposite side of that coin is also true. Many people feel *sssoooo* in control in all areas of their lives *except* with food. Again, the same solution works: Let go of the need to control in other areas of life and you will free up more energy to be in control of what you eat.

Remember, *control is an illusion.* Anyone with children will affirm that! The **need** to control is often rampant in overweight people. Much time and effort are spent trying to control people and situations that there's little energy left to control oneself. And that is the only true control there is: self-control.

·· o ··

Å *I have complete control over my emotions.*

Å *I gladly discard foods and belongings I no longer need.*

> *I am a great believer in luck.*
> *I find the harder I work,*
> *The more of it I have.*
> — Thomas Jefferson

Å *I actively seek exercise and enjoy a very healthy body.*

My associate and dear friend, Nan Bolomey, uses the following equation often. I love it and share it with you here:

$$E + P = O$$

It means *Event* plus *Perception* equals *Outcome*. You may not be able to control the events in your life but once they happen, how you *choose* to perceive them will dictate your experience of the event—your Outcome. If, for example, your boss yells at you, you can choose to believe that s/he thinks you're worthless and go have a big cheeseburger to soothe your hurt feelings. Or you could choose to believe that s/he had an big family argument that morning and you just happen to be in the wrong place at the wrong time and are the subject of misdirected anger and let it roll off your shoulders. In other words, *you don't take it personally*. Or you could choose an infinite number of other possibilities, none of which has anything to do with you! How would you rather live your life—outside in or inside out? Believe me, the latter is preferable.

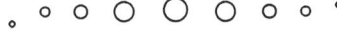

Å   *I am wonderfully worthy of giving and receiving unconditional love.*

Å   *I am always on time and love the feeling of being on time.*

Å   *I am blessed with good and exciting friends.*

Å   *I always think of new affirmations very easily. I truly believe in the power of my affirmations.*

Read *Think and Grow Rich* by Napoleon Hill.

The only thing you have control over is your mind and when you choose to exercise that control you will be among the most powerful people on the planet. You will be able to control every outcome of every experience in your life. Sound like fun? It is!

According to author and lecturer, Marianne Williamson, the definition of a miracle is a "shift in perception." Want to make some miracles today? You now know how.

Many overweight people hate their jobs (yes, there is a correlation between job satisfaction and weight). If you do, there's a number of actions you can take to resolve that problem. The two most obvious are: 1) change your job, or 2) change your mind.

BUSY WORK

Never hide behind busy work. It takes just as much energy to fail as it does to succeed. You must constantly guard against the trap of falling into a routine of remaining busy with unimportant chores that will provide you with an excuse to avoid meaningful challenges or opportunities that could change your life for the better.

Your hours are your most precious possession.
This day is all you have.
Waste not a minute.
NEVER HIDE BEHIND BUSY WORK.

from *The Spellbinder's Gift*
by Og Mandino

> **ACTION**
> *The superior man is modest in his speech,*
> *but excels in his actions.*
> — Confucius

Don't fixate or obsess on a particular goal weight. Give yourself a 10-pound range. Your weight fluctuates daily, often depending on salt intake the day before. Allow your body to find where it wants to be. It's more important that you look and feel good and that your clothes fit comfortably than some arbitrary number on a piece of equipment that's probably broken!

At what point will you be "good enough"? Believe me, being good enough has little to do with your weight. If you're not good enough now, losing weight **will not** make you so.

Your world is a reflection of your belief about your world. If you think the world is an unsafe place (remember, one of the most powerful dynamics of the subconscious is to keep you safe—often under layers of fat) often you will have unsafe events show up in your life. Remember the "thinker" and the "prover."

> *Many things which cannot be overcome*
> *when they are together,*
> *yield themselves up*
> *when taken little by little.*
> — Plutarch

In King Arthur's time, "sin" meant to "miss the mark" during archery competition. To sin means that you made a mistake. So you practice and get better and get closer to your ideal behavior.

How often do you create a crisis so you can eat about it?

Repeat the following sentence to yourself then close your eyes, go inside and get your mind's response to it: "**I am 100% accountable for everything in my life—with *no* blame.**" This is a very liberating belief. There is no blame to assess because your life is made up of a series of lessons. You can choose to learn them quickly or more slowly. If you choose to learn them more slowly, they will present themselves to you until you learn them. No mistakes, no blame, just lessons.

Everybody grew up in a dysfunctional family. Let it go. You are now an adult.

> **MISTAKES**
> *There are no mistakes.*
> *The events we bring upon ourselves,*
> *no matter how unpleasant,*
> *Are necessary in order to learn*
> *what we need to learn*
> *whatever steps we take,*
> *they're necessary to reach the places*
> *we've chosen to go.*
> — John Dewey

Today, change your mind about how you've been perceiving something and create a more pleasant reality for yourself.

Å *I awaken each morning relaxed and refreshed and full of energy.*

Today, practice detachment. Step back from yourself and any situation you're in and observe it as though you were not involved. Do this without judgment. Most thoughts we have are judgments, so this will be an interesting exercise. Practice judging less and less critically until you can just observe.

One way to minimize your inclination to be judgmental—especially about yourself—is to meditate. According to Deepak Chopra, it's the only time that you're awake and not judging. You can then take this ability into your waking life and practice it more easily.

Negativity is very heavy. It weighs you down. Listen to yourself. How negative are you? If you don't want to **be** it, don't think it or say it. It's how you start reversing the negative spiral in which most of us live.

Å *My body is perfect, and I love it and treat it very well.*

Å *I love being a very positive and powerful person.*

Å *I enjoy my dreams, remember them, and use them for personal insight and for recreation.*

Read *You'll See It When You Believe It* by Wayne Dyer.

I was a guest on a radio show and the first caller was very angry with me. He accused me of being a charlatan (despite my credentials which had been given at the top of the show) and of just trying to make money from the pain of others. I chose to be kind and gentle in the face of his rage, knowing what would happen next. For the next two hours callers supported me and hypnosis (we **do** love an underdog!). I chose to believe that his wife had just run off with a hypnotherapist. Now, obviously, I had no way of knowing his agenda. I just chose a belief that supported the outcome I wanted—not to take it personally.

Several months later, I received a call from him apologizing for his behavior. It seems his wife was morbidly obese and dying from it, and she was unwilling or unable to stop herself from dying, so he had to take his anger out on somebody. You see, you never know until you know. I was very glad I'd been kind to him.

Breathe!

Love is behavior.

What are you allowing yourself to be victimized by? And how much is it causing you to "eat about it"?

How do you use your wounds like childhood traumas, for example, as weapons—to manipulate and control others? Or to give you one more excuse to eat when you're not hungry? Do you know it's killing you? Grow up and begin being in charge of your life.

Å   *I love to drink water and drink at least 8 glasses a day.*

Life is not supposed to be a struggle.

Definition of a healthy relationship: Long periods of peace, followed by conflict, followed by conflict resolution, followed by long periods of peace.

Å *I am in an extremely healthy, happy and fulfilling relationship.*

Å *I love myself.*
Other people love me.
My parents love me.
I love my parents.
My family loves me.
I love my family.
The people I work with love me.
I love the people I work with.
I have lots of friends who love me.
People love to be with me.

I really love myself.

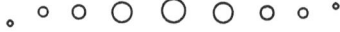

Many problems will solve themselves if you leave them alone. Your mission is to know which need your help and which don't.

Peace and calm are not the same as boredom.

○

Human beings are by nature problem-solvers. However often when we don't have one to solve, we'll *create* one! Then, of course, eat about it!

○

Albert Einstein postulated many years ago that if we took every human being on the planet and condensed us down into solid matter, that matter would be about the size of an aspirin tablet! How much time do you spend thinking about your body which basically doesn't exist?

∘ ○ ○ ◯ ◯ ◯ ○ ∘ °

Å *I love the feeling of my soft, smooth skin.*

Å *All unnecessary fat now freely and easily leaves my body.*

○

You've all heard the saying that the body is the temple of the soul. What that means is that my Soul or Spirit is more powerful than I can even imagine but can only be as powerful as its vessel. To allow your spirit more power, it is imperative that your body be as healthy as possible. As you get physically healthier, you will also become spiritually more powerful.

Our deepest fear is not
> that we are inadequate.
Our deepest fear is that
> we are powerful beyond measure.

It is our light, not our darkness,
> that most frightens us.
We ask ourselves, who am I to be brilliant,
> georgeous, talented.
Actually, who are you not to be? . . .

Your playing small does not serve the world.
There's nothing enlightened
> about shrinking so other people
> > won't feel insecure around you . . .

As we are liberated from
> our own fear,
Our presence automatically liberates others.

> — *Nelson Mandela*
> *1994 Inaugural Speech*

Buy organic fruits and vegetables whenever possible. They save your liver the effort of cleansing the toxins from your body. Our livers were meant to work about 8 hours a day. Most of ours are going full-tilt for 24 hours.

○

Meditate 20 minutes a day. It's about 1/100th of your day. I am very results oriented. I meditate because *it works*. After my meditations, I always do things that save time or produce greater results. I find myself doing things right the first time which always *saves at least 20 minutes!* I once asked my friend Joel if he meditates. He said brusquely, "No," then followed that with, "Oh, I sit quietly for 20 minutes every day." Call it what you want, just do it. If you have trouble quieting your mind, listen to a hypnosis tape.

Meditation gets you in touch with your intuition. Watch what wonderful things happen in your life when you expand your intuition.

○

Stephen Levine, author and lecturer and expert on death and dying, says, "If you walked into a restaurant and sat in a booth next to two people who were talking to each other as mercilessly as you talk to yourself, you'd have to leave. It would make you so sick, you wouldn't be able to eat." Yet we treat ourselves this badly with little regard for our own feelings. Show a little mercy on yourself. You're doing the best you can. If you could do better, you would do better.

○

Å   *Negative thoughts of eating do not enter my mind.*

Think about how you might feel if, on your deathbed, you looked back and had regrets over the many things you didn't do because you were going to do them when . . . "I lose 20 pounds" or . . . "I make more money" or . . . "when the kids finish school" or . . . or . . . or—it could go on and on. **Get your life off hold now.** Do something—anything—that you've been putting off.

○

Stop being "Captain of the World."

○

Dear Friend:

I appreciate all the help you've been giving me lately but it's really not necessary. That's my job.

Love,
God

○

This is a tip from Scott Adams, creator of the "Dilbert" comic strip:

Write down what one goal 15 times each day. Do it until you reach that goal. Even if you're skeptical. Be as precise as you'd like. Do it until you get it.

Å   *I have the power to stop myself.*
    I eat only as much food as my body requires.

I believe one primary function of affirmations is to get you in touch with how powerful you really are. An affirmation is a statement of truth in advance.

○

It is self-abuse to overfeed your body.

Look at all the baggage you've been carrying around all these years: old wounds, grudges, resentments, anger, hurt. How are they serving you to keep carrying them? Isn't it time to put them down?

○

How do you use your wounds as weapons to manipulate others?

○

TELL THE TRUTH (to yourself).

○ ○ ○ ○ ○ ○ ○ ○

When you caretake others you deprive them of the opportunity of living life for themselves.

○

Å *My attitude, my appearance, my general health, the way I dress, everything improves daily.*

Give from your excess, not from your substance. I equate it to principal and interest in the bank. If I give away my principal, there's less there to grow interest. If I give from my interest, I keep my principal growing more interest.

This especially goes for your work. Women in particular are more apt to give and give and give at work. I had a job once and I noticed that the men *always* left for lunch and most of the women worked through lunch. Don't do it. If you haven't got your health you won't have a job anyway. Besides, do you know what most corporations do with you when you burn out? They throw you away! In the words of the late, great George Burns, "I've visited many friends on their deathbeds and *not one* of them ever said 'I wished I'd spent more time at the office.'"

This lesson was brought home very clearly to me again by my dear friend, Joel Junker. When his young wife was dying of cancer, they made the conscious choice that he should continue rowing (he'd rowed at Cambridge and fell in love with the sport). The reason was obvious: He needed to maintain his health. He was no good to either of them if he, too, got sick. This was a man in a new law practice working to support his family financially as well as be there for his terminally ill wife. If he could find time to exercise, you certainly can too.

○

If you have a problem with someone, *it's not their problem— it's yours.*

Detachment is one of the most powerful tools you can learn. Don't take it all so personally.

○

All tears are healing tears.

Have you ever asked yourself 'What does s/he see in him/her"? We are unconscious about most of the reasons why we are attracted to the people to whom we are attracted. The more you know about yourself (*with no blame*), the more accountable you will be and the better choices you will make.

The whole world is your student; the whole world is your teacher.

> *If you still believe in coincidences . . . you're not paying attention!*
> — Richard Bach

Å ***I have the right to say no to food, because I like myself and others like me too.***

Å ***The only reason to eat is for the health and integrity of my body. Losing weight builds a strong, healthy body and builds my self-esteem and acceptance. Losing weight means being a winner, and I am a winner.***

Å ***I live a glorious, fear-free life. There is nothing to fear in life.***

If you haven't set up verbal and emotional boundaries, your body will give you a physical one.

Read *Getting the Love You Want* by Harville Hendrix.

Hendrix says that we attract partners into our lives to help us heal childhood wounds. However, if we stay unconscious about it we end up repeating those wounds. You attract those who can **help** you. Know it and you can achieve it. Otherwise, you'll divorce and remarry—the same person. Different name, different face, different job, but the same person. And you'll probably continue bitching and eating about it. Aren't you tired of it?

According to Hendrix, every married couple, whether married 5 or 50 years, has only three to five arguments. And they have these for the rest of their lives. And, if they're unconscious about them, they may perceive themselves as fighting a lot (and often eating about it!). If you're married, sit down with your partner and write down what you each think those three to five arguments are. Talk about them and resolve them or *agree to disagree* about them or get counseling about them. Just bring them to the fore, talk about them and be conscious of them. They're not nearly so intimidating when you bring them into the light.

○

The definition of stress: An organism's reaction to change. That's it. Doesn't sound so terrible, does it? However, the latest medical research is giving more and more credence to the effects of stress on heart disease. I find it fascinating that change is the only guarantee in life and most of us fight it tooth and nail. When you learn how to adapt easily to change, you will significantly decrease your need to eat because of it.

○

Read *Conversations with God* by Neale Donald Walsch.
I always wake up smiling when I read a page or two the night before.

The best and the worst news you can receive:
"This too shall pass"

It takes three lies to cover up one lie. Many people lie when it would be just as easy to tell the truth. Lying is very stressful. Don't lie. And there's another thing you don't have to eat about.

> **"PERFECTION"**
> *The "C" students run the world.*
> — Harry S. Truman

Perfectionists aren't nourished by praise—because they don't believe it.

Perfectionism is boring. It keeps you stuck where you are ("No use trying—I can't do it perfectly anyway").

> **FAILURE**
> *It's good to fail now and again—*
> *you learn a lot more out of failure*
> *than you do out of success.*
> — Ian Hunter

Don't analyze too much. Change happens in the body. Analyzing keeps it in your head. You will never have enough information. Studies show that people who try more things fail at more things and also succeed at more things. People who try few things fail less frequently, yet succeed less frequently too.

DON'T BE AFRAID TO FAIL

You've failed many times.
*   Although you don't remember.*
You fell down the first time
*   you tried to walk.*
You almost drowned the
*   first time you tried to swim.*
Did you hit the ball the first
*   time you swung a bat?*
Heavy hitters, the ones who
*   hit the most home runs, also*
*   strike out a lot.*
R.H. Macy failed seven times
*   before his store in New York caught on.*
English novelist John Creasey got 753 rejection slips
*   before he published 564 books.*
Babe Ruth struck out 1,330 times
*   but he also hit 714 home runs.*
Don't worry about failure
Worry about the chances you miss
*   when you don't even try.*

                              (author unknown)

Å *My mind is open; my body is relaxed and at ease.*

Å *I feel better than I have in years.*

The fears I have about letting go of my excess weight are:

_____

_____

_____

_____

_____

_____

_____

> **FEAR**
> *Fear comes from uncertainty.*
> *When we are absolutely certain,*
> *whether of our worth or worthlessness,*
> *we are almost impervious to fear.*
> — William Congreve

"There is no fear here"

When you stay present you'll find your fears dissipating quickly. Fear often occurs when contemplating tomorrow with today's brain.

Read *Feel the Fear and Do it Anyway* by Susan Jeffers. There's a wonderful mantra from that book:

When you feel yourself becoming fearful about something, simply tell yourself, "I'll handle it." Because you usually have.

The number one reason people don't have the things in their lives that they say they want is that, on some level, they don't believe they deserve them. What's missing in your life? What beliefs may you be holding that affirm a belief that you don't deserve it/them?

Right now you have the life you believe you deserve.

If you want to know what you believe, look at your life. It is a reflection on what you hold to be the truth. Is it hard and mistrusting and scary? Then that's what you hold to be true about life. Or is it easy, abundant, and basically happy? To change your life, change your mind *first*.

> *Genius begins great works,*
> *Labor alone finishes it.*
> — Joseph Joubert

Å **All parts of my body, mind and emotions are working in complete harmony. My vision is bright and distinct.**

Being in "victim" sounds like this: "It's not my fault" . . . (that the donut was in the kitchen, that my friend cooked this food so I had to eat it . . .)

○ ○ ○ ○ ○ ○ ○ ○

How many of you ever got five A's and one B on your report card? Which grade got the attention? No wonder it's so easy for most of us to be negative!

There's only three uses your body has for food:

1. It can use it for energy, fuel and cellular replacement.
2. It can slough it off as waste.
3. It can store it *as fat.*

Your body can convert any food into fat. The myth is that if you don't want to *be* fat, don't *eat* fat. Your body doesn't have to convert fat to store it. That's why it's so easy for it to store the excess fat you eat. However, it *will* store *any* food that you eat which cannot readily be used or excreted. That's why quantity is just as important as quality of food you eat.

Dr. Wayne Dyer has a wonderful antidote for worry (and how often do we eat about worry?). Just ask yourself one question: "Can I do anything about it?". If you can, *do it.* If you can't, let it go! Sounds simple, huh? Practice, practice, practice!

A study was done several years ago that revealed about 93% of what we worry about *never even happens!* Just think about how much time and energy we waste on *nothing!*

Have you noticed that life always seems to work out *whether or not you worry about it.* Seems like you could save yourself a lot of time and energy by not worrying so much.

What you focus your attention on is what your unconscious mind will attract to you and will create in your life. What are you giving your attention to? If you knew how powerful your thoughts were, you would be very vigilant with them.

Get a pedicure.

> **POTENTIAL**
> *Life itself is a race, marked by a start, and a finish.*
> *It is what we learn during the race,*
> *and how we apply it, that determines whether*
> *our participation has had a particular value.*
> *If we learn from each success, and each failure, and*
> *improve ourselves through the process, then, at the end,*
> *we have fulfilled our potential and performed well.*
> — Dr. F. Porsche

A study was done recently in Texas, then replicated in England, which compared prescription antidepressants with St. John's Wort, a ground cover plant found all over northwestern United States, among other locales. The St. John's Wort worked better than nothing (control group) and equally as well as the prescription drugs in alleviating depressive symptoms. You can find it at any health food store. It is *imperative* that you consult your physician prior to taking it and that you *do not, under any circumstances take St. John's Wort with prescription antidepressants. The combination could kill you.*

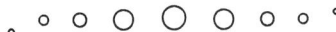

Å   *My hearing is excellent.*
    My mind is sharp and my memory is strong.

Å   *My heart is normal, calm, and very strong.*
    My stomach digests food with ease.

Å   *My eyes are bright and clear.*
    I see and hear perfectly.

PMS

Women can experience PMS in varying degrees for up to two weeks out of the month. Let's look at that. If you gain 3 pounds when you're premenstrual and then after you start your period, lose 2 pounds, that's just a 1 pound net weight gain as a result of PMS. Doesn't sound too bad. That's just 12 pounds a year. That's just 120 pounds in 10 years! *Just from PMS eating.* That doesn't take into account all the other reasons we eat. There are many antidotes to PMS symptoms. Among my favorites are:

- Walk 20 minutes a day. Studies show that many women with severe cases of PMS have levels of serotonin which are minuscule. This is the hormone in the body which is produced from sunlight and exercise which make you feel good. Seratonin is made from carbohydrates in the absence of sun and exercise.

- Take 200 mg of vitamin B6 daily. You'll be amazed at the reduction of PMS symptoms. Your period may actually sneak up on you.

There's a variety of homeopathic remedies. Check them out at your health food store. They often work differently for different people.

- Try Rescue Remedy® or Nature's Rescue® available at many health stores. As well as reducing stress and lowering resistance to losing weight, it acts as a calmative during PMS.

- Eliminate refined sugar and Nutrasweet® from your diet. If you have trouble doing this, try 200 mcg of chromium picolinate a day.

- Listen to a meditation or hypnosis tape 20 minutes a day. This quiet time helps many of your internal processes return to normal.

One of the by-products of stress is too much adrenaline in your system. This has been linked to the deterioration of organs (like your heart).

There are three ways adrenaline is eliminated from your system:

- Minute amounts are dissipated through emotional tears.
- Minute amounts are dissipated through meditation.
- By far the largest amounts of adrenaline are metabolized by large muscle activity.

The largest muscles in your body are in your thighs and your seat. You know what I'm going to say—go for a walk. It physiologically reduces your stress.

When you don't have the time to go for a walk is when you absolutely, positively *must* go for a walk.

Exercise prevents bone deterioration. Women, if you're taking calcium to forestall osteoporosis when your bodies cease producing estrogen, you must do weight-bearing exercise. That's what gets calcium into the bones. Otherwise it could collect in your kidneys and cause medical problems there later in life—as well as the osteoporosis you sought to avoid.

A recent study was being done with over 20,000 nurses on the effects of calcium in reducing cholesterol. The study had to be terminated when it was found that the nurses taking the calcium had such a radical drop in their cholesterol that the researchers could not in good conscience continue the study and deprive the control group of such great benefits. Take your calcium—1,000 to 1,500 mg. per day for women. An easy way to get it is in Tums® (or an equivalent). Just be sure there's no aluminum in whatever product you choose. Then go for a walk.

Exercise produces high-density lipoproteins (HDLs)—the "good" cholesterol. HDLs help eliminate low-density lipoproteins (LDLs—the "bad" cholesterol) from your body.

Take the stairs instead of the elevator. A friend of mine worked on the 35th floor of an office building. She took the elevator to the 30th floor and walked the rest of the way. The following week she took the elevator to the 29th floor. Each week she took the elevator to one less floor. She got a great workout and had the time to do it!

You burn more calories standing than sitting; you burn more calories walking than standing; you burn more calories running than walking. Just do something.

Look at how our modern technology supports not moving. The "clapper" to turn on lights; the garage door opener; blenders and food processors; bread machines (remember kneading bread—it took energy!), and the ultimate "wuss machine" the remote control!

When you hear the resistance in your head (it often sounds like, "I don't have time"), acknowledge it, and then **move your body** anyway. You have the time. Think of it this way: exercise creates more energy in your body to do whatever it is you need to do—***in less time***. It also adds ***years*** to your life—that's time. That's priceless time.

Å *My thighs are muscular.*

Å *All of the weight I lose will stay off.*

Å *I have peace of mind, love, joy, and self-confidence.*

Å *All parts of my body function perfectly.*

Å *I am calm and relaxed and in control of what I eat.*

Read *Diet for a New America* by John Robbins.

Å **Losing weight is highly pleasing to me.**

Å **I am always thinking and come up with great new ideas.**

Å **My body is great.**

> **IMAGINATION**
> *Five minutes, just before going to sleep,*
> *given to a bit of directed imagination*
> *regarding achievement possibilities of the morrow,*
> *will steadily and increasingly bear fruit,*
> *particularly if all ideas of difficulty, worry*
> *or fear are resolutely ruled out and replaced*
> *by those of accomplishment and smiling courage.*
> — Frederick Pierce

You are limited only by your imagination and your belief in what is possible. What *is* possible?

RECOMMENDED READING LIST

OBESITY AND DYSFUNCTIONAL FAMILIES

1. *Weight, Sex and Marriage: A Delicate Balance.* Richard B. Stuart and Barbara Jacobson. W. W. Norton & Co., 1987.

2. *Diets Don't Work.* Robert Schwartz. Breakthrough Publishing, 1984.

3. **Fat is a Family Affair.* Judi Hollis. Harper & Row, 1985.

4. **Feeding the Empty Heart: Adult Children and Compulsive Eating.* Barbara McFarland and Tyeis Baker-Baumann. Harper & Row, 1988.

5. **Take It Off and Keep It Off.* Anonymous. Contemporary Books Inc., Chicago, 1984.

6. **Recovery from Compulsive Behavior: How To Transcend Your Troubled Family.* Lane Lasater, Ph.D. Health Communication, Inc., 1988.

7. **Willpower Is Not Enough: Recovering from Addictions of Every Kind.* A. Washton and D. Boundy. Harper Perennial, 1988.

8. *Keeping It Off.* R. H. Colvin and S. C. Olson. KIO, 18 Hillcrest Dr., Carbondale, Illinois.

9. *When Food Is Love.* Geneen Roth. N.A.L.

---

* Especially pertinent for adult children of alcoholics who also have a weight problem.

DYSFUNCTIONAL FAMILY SYSTEMS IN GENERAL

1. *Homecoming.* John Bradshaw. Bantam Books.

2. *Healing the Shame that Binds You.* John Bradshaw. Health Communication Inc.

3. *Bradshaw: On the Family.* John Bradshaw. Health Communication Inc.

4. *Choice Making: For Co-Dependents, Adult Children, and Spirituality Seekers.* Sharon Wegscheider-Cruse, 1985.

5. *Adult Children: Secrets of the Dysfunctional Family.* J. Friel, 1988.

6. *Co-Dependent No More.* Melody Beattie. Hazelden. 1987.

7. *Adult Children of Alcoholics.* Janet Geringer Woititz. Health Communication, 1983.

8. *Language of Letting Go.* Melody Beattie. HarperCollins.

9. *Healing the Child Within.* Charles L. Whitfield, M.D. Health Communications, 1987.

10. *Dance of Anger.* Harriet Lerner. HarperCollins.